SEVERE DEPRESSION

THE ESSENTIAL GUIDE FOR CARERS

Tony Frais, MA

Published by
Anthony Frais
9 Sandhill Oval
Leeds LS17 8EB

afrais@tiscali.co.uk

ISBN 978 0 95 48068 4 2

Contents

Acknowledgements

I would like to thank the following people for their helpful suggestions in the preparation of this booklet.

Professor Linda Gask, Professor of Primary Care Psychiatry, University of Manchester.

Dr. Elaine McNichol, Academic lead for Service Users and Carers at the School of Healthcare, University of Leeds.

Ruth Hannan, Policy and Development Manager (mental health) at Carers Trust.

FOREWORD

This excellent guide leads the reader through the different stages of the carer's and patient's journey through the experience of severe depression. The guide balances empathy with the challenges they are facing alongside clarity about what to expect and practical strategies for managing situations as they arise. There are key messages about the importance of the carer looking after their own health and well being in order to be able to support the patient and work in partnership with them to overcome severe depression.

It is an honest insight underpinned by the author's own experiences and whilst the emphasis is on the carer, it is a guide that is equally valuable to the patient themselves and their wider family and friends in facilitating an understanding of the experience of severe depression.

Elaine McNichol
Academic Lead for Service User and Carer Involvement
University of Leeds

INTRODUCTION

This booklet has been designed to help those caring for someone with severe depression. You may not describe yourself as a carer, you may be the depressed person's spouse, sibling, parent, child or friend. The term carer is used in the broadest sense as someone who is offering support and care to someone experiencing severe depression.

Severe depression is a seriously disabling illness affecting 5% of the population. But it is not only the depressed person with a problem. The effects of the illness also impacts on the person's carers. Carers are suddenly thrust in to caring for a person suffering from an illness they barely understand. The carer begins to lead a life which can at times be overwhelming and demanding. Normal social and family life can be disrupted. As the illness progresses, many carers report feelings of being worn down physically and mentally from the stress of caring as well as not being able to plan for the future. They also experience a sense of hopelessness, frustration, annoyance and feel neglected and isolated. As a result of this, there is the danger that carers could also become depressed.

But caring for a severely depressed person may not necessarily be a negative experience in every case. Carers can and do find a positive meaning to their role and are able to achieve a purposeful, rewarding and effective quality of care which can not only benefit the depressed person but can also lead to reduced levels of stress for the carer.

So the issue is just how can carers best deal with the situation they suddenly find themselves in; what the future holds and how they can best help the depressed person and themselves.

As someone caring for a person with severe depression, you will be faced with seeing them through their illness. However, it is also important to think about your own well-being.

Each part of this booklet describes the significant stages of the carer's and depressed person's journey through the experience of severe depression.

The booklet includes the thoughts of real life carers and severely depressed people who best capture their emotions at points of time during the course of the illness.

Throughout this booklet, the carer and the severely depressed person are considered as partners who are facing this experience together.

Part 1 The nature of severe depression
As a first step towards successful caring, it is important that the carer has a good understanding of the nature of severe depression and how it affects the person.

Part 2 The impact of severe depression on carers
This section discusses how the first experiences of looking after a severely depressed person may begin to have an impact on your life.

Part 3 Seeking help and support
How carers can begin to seek the help and support they need.

Part 4 Stigma and seeking treatment
This discusses how the stigma of severe depression can often be a barrier to the people seeking treatment.

Part 5 Visiting the GP
This section details what you might experience when the severely depressed person agrees to visit their GP. Although many patients are happy to have someone with them at their GP consultation, some patients may be unwilling to involve the carer. The GP has a duty of confidentiality to the patient. The issues regarding the medication prescribed by the GP are also discussed.

Part 6 The treatment resistant patient
Research has shown that approximately 35% of severely depressed patients respond to antidepressant medication prescribed by their GP. But for the majority, the first choice of antidepressant may not result in a significant reduction of symptoms. If the patient still does not improve after switching to a different antidepressant, they may be considered as being treatment resistant. The patient now enters what is known as secondary care and is referred to a consultant psychiatrist. However, success in finding new and effective medication from the psychiatrist is not guaranteed. This may be the most difficult time for both carer and patient.

Part 7 Recovery and relapse prevention
Recovery from severe depression marks a time which is just as crucial as at any time during the course of the illness for both carer and patient. A large percentage of patients remain vulnerable to relapses. In order to lessen the chances

of relapses, it is important that the patient receives ongoing treatment such as psychotherapy in addition to remaining on the medication.

Part 8 Care for the carer
How you can access advice and support in order to protect your own health and well-being.

Part 9 The positives of caring
Despite the stresses and difficulties, caring can turn out to be a positive experience.

Key points to remember

Useful websites for advice and support

References

PART 1 THE NATURE OF SEVERE DEPRESSION

As a carer, you will be better prepared to face the challenges ahead if you have a good understanding of the nature of the illness. Understanding severe depression will help you cope with the changes in the person's behaviour and reactions.

The experience and attitudes to suffering from severe depression inevitably varies between different people However, there are a number of common threads in terms of symptoms. The Royal College of Psychiatrist's leaflet 'Working in Partnership with Psychiatrists and Carers,' lists the following symptoms which if continuing for more than a few weeks, indicates a severe depressive episode.

Changes in the person's behaviour
As a carer, you may notice that the person:
- is unhappy most of the time
- has lost confidence in themselves
- expresses feelings of guilt, shame and worthlessness
- is irritable and, perhaps angry
- is tearful
- has lost their appetite, or eats more than usual
- has changed their sleeping pattern
- is extremely tired
- has problems concentrating
- looks and feels anxious
- is withdrawn and has lost interest in life, including sex
- isn't looking after themselves as well as usual
- feeling suicidal

Episodes of severe depression can last an average of four to eight months but there can be cases where it can last for longer. Severe depression is different from mild to moderate depression. The causes of mild to moderate depression can, generally speaking, be more easily identified as a direct result of personal difficulties such as the loss of a loved one, mounting financial difficulties and unemployment. It can also be the result of suffering a physical illness such as heart attack, diabetes or cancer.

Severe depression may at times have roots which stem from these catastrophic life events but it is also a case of increasing negativity about life in general. People who are heading for severe depression often miss the clues such as a loss of enjoyment in doing the things they liked to do and a growing uncertainty about their future prospects in life. These feelings may be dismissed by the person as no more than just being a bit fed up with things and nothing more serious than that.

However, this insidious build up of increasingly negative and sometimes irrational thinking and action begins to undermine and adversely affect the person's normal character and personality which can lead to the descent into severe depression. When this happens, and it can sometimes happen very suddenly, it leaves the person frightened and bewildered; they cannot understand what is happening to them and why.

Severe depression is an experience which is almost impossible to compare with any physical illness. Severely depressed people often become frustrated at not being able to adequately convey to family and friends just what a terrible experience it is. The depressed person becomes suspended in time; there is no past, there is no future, just a day by day experience of a mostly miserable and almost unbearable existence.

Severely depressed people may have difficulty managing everyday affairs; lack a sense of meaning in life, have few goals or aims, lack sense of direction. They are likely to become uninterested with life, feel unable to develop new attitudes or behaviours.[1]

Although not a serious symptom, there is another feature shared by most severely depressed people in that their recollection of past personal memories can tend to be rather vague and lacking in detail; they may struggle to recall happier times from the past.

Despite initial urging from friends and family, it is impossible for the severely depressed person to just 'snap out of it.' For many people, this locked in pattern of misery cannot be changed by such things as going on a luxury holiday or winning some money on the lottery.

Nothing highlights the depths of the suffering more than the fact that almost without exception, severely depressed people at some point think of suicide as a way out of their misery. Thoughts of suicide can often be the significant difference between severe depression and mild to moderate cases.

Anxiety

A high percentage of severely depressed people have high levels of anxiety. This is a significant and important feature which needs to be understood in order to develop a more complete picture of the nature of severe depression. It is widely accepted that anxiety and severe depression go hand in hand. Anxiety causes an increased level of stress hormones such as adrenaline into the bloodstream resulting in a feeling which is sometimes described as having butterflies in the stomach. This effect contributes to making severe depression a physically uncomfortable illness in addition to the adverse psychological effects.

Diurnal variations – the false recovery

There is an unusual and not well understood aspect to the nature of severe depression. This is the phenomenon of diurnal variations. Diurnal means something which happens on a daily basis. A daily variation in mood has been recognized as a characteristic feature of severe depression. The severely depressed person who experiences diurnal variations typically experiences low mood in the morning but mood improves towards the evening and there are cases where mood is better in the morning and becoming worse in the evening. During these periods, the person may believe they have finally overcome the illness However, this 'recovery' is often a false dawn and the full weight of the symptoms invariably returns the next day. There may be cases where a 'recovery' of this type can last for a few days but again, symptoms return much to the disappointment of the depressed person.

PART 2 THE IMPACT OF SEVERE DEPRESSION ON CARERS

Most carers are completely unprepared for living and coping with a person suffering from severe depression. The fact that severe depression is a mysterious and complex illness which cannot be easily explained or described makes it difficult for both the carer and the depressed person to convey to others what they are experiencing. It is also an illness that some people may think trivial and you may find that family and friends may not fully appreciate the impact it is having on your life.

If the person continues to exhibit symptoms of severe depression for more than two weeks, it is likely that they are severely depressed. However, the most significant symptom of severe depression is when the person begins to talk to you about feeling suicidal.

Severely depressed people may talk openly about feeling suicidal. However, during these early stages of the illness, it is possible that this may be another way in which the person is trying to convey to the carer the depth of the suffering. However, any talk of suicide should not be taken lightly. Circumstances where there may be a more serious risk of suicide and what can be done are discussed in Part 6.

As the illness progresses, other distressing aspects for carers include: being upset by the depressed person's irritability and lack of interest, feeling discouraged by an increasing sense of hopelessness and concerns about their future. Social life also begins to be affected.

'She didn't want to go out, so we didn't go out. We'd knock back invitations ... then they stopped coming, so we stayed home.'[2]

Expressing concern to the depressed person that they are behaving in a way which is not like their normal selves and a concern that something is wrong is often a useful first step. This signifies to them that there is a genuine desire to try and understand what is going on; what they are thinking about and why. The intention is to make it clear that you are an active partner and willing to give all the help and support in overcoming the illness.

One study describes the experience of caring for a severely depressed person and the impact it had on the life of the carer. Many carers reported feelings of anxiety and exhaustion.

'There is constant emotional tension ... everyday I wake up and think — What is going to happen today, what will they be like?'

'You come home from work, you get changed and you're on. It's like working double shifts.'

'You have to be ever-vigilant ... everyday there is a potential crisis.'

'You live each day feeling like you're walking on eggshells.' I didn't know what to say to him, to make him feel better. But I was also afraid of saying anything at all because any little thing could have made him feel worse.'

'You can only keep propping the other person up for so long, then you feel deflated and exhausted ... and then you start to feel down.'[3]

Another issue which you may experience is there may be a lack of positive feedback as to whether your contribution and efforts are being appreciated. There may also be times when you feel upset because the severely depressed person may take out their anger and frustration on you. However, it is important to remember that this hostility is more a result of the illness and not their normal personality.

Although you may make every effort to comfort them, the nature of severe depression is such that there will be times when they may simply want to be left alone for a period of time as one depressed person found:

'The way I look at it, if you care for a person, you've got to let them be who they want to be at that time. If they want to talk, they talk. If they don't want to talk, they don't talk. If they just want to sit there and stare into space, but as long as you are there for them'[3]

Communication
As the illness progresses, normal conversation between you and the person may begin to break down. As one person explained:

'It is not the relationship that existed prior to the illness ... So the things that you talk about in a relationship which are around plans for the future ... about the children and where you might go on holiday or ... what's happening in the world or what's happened today. You don't have any of those conversations, because the person with the depression has no interest in those conversations ... So actually it's a very lonely period.'[3]

18

Achieving effective communication as soon as possible between yourself and the severely depressed person is important. The ability to be open with one another, share feelings and thoughts can be one of the keys to success. But achieving meaningful communication may not be easy. If you do not have early success, there is the danger that you may become frustrated and may feel less inclined in trying to communicate with them. However, these difficulties can be overcome.

In the first instance, you need to be aware that severely depressed people often have a short attention span which means effective communication may only be possible in frequent but brief conversations. However, there will also be times when symptoms are so severe that they will find it almost impossible to talk. The timing of communication between you and the depressed person is therefore crucial.

When symptoms become less severe and they seem to be more approachable, this could be the time to have a more relaxed conversation. Severely depressed people may find that having the ability to talk to you about their feelings in a meaningful way can be emotionally beneficial. As one person describes:

'Talking gets my frustrations and anger out ... It takes a load off ... it calms me down ... You're not quite so on your own. You don't feel quite so isolated. I think you just come out of your hole a bit.'[3]

Being able to talk to the depressed person without being judged and criticized will be appreciated. But what effective communication can also do is to establish that both of you are on the same side; a united effort with the aim of overcoming the illness.

Family and friends
Inevitably, family and close friends become aware that there are problems and with the best intentions, they may want to try and help as best they can. However, there are challenges to overcome.

You are likely to be faced with trying to describe what the severely depressed person is going through. They are also likely to be mystified by the situation.

As some carers explain:

'they just don't know how to handle it... it's not their fault, you can't blame them...'[3]

'People are ignorant about mental illness; they don't understand it. They can sympathize or empathize with a caregiver for someone with cancer or dementia or a stroke, but they just don't get mental illness. They don't appreciate how difficult it is to be in this position.'[4]

Can the support of family and friends make a difference? They can certainly be a great help if they have a good understanding of what the depressed person is going through in order to provide the right emotional and sympathetic support; it is important to demonstrate that they care, listen in a non judgemental way and be prepared to keep what they see and hear confidential. The depressed person may appreciate this support because family and friends can sometimes give a fresh perspective on the situation in addition to the sole voice of the carer. Encouraging family support can also be helpful to your mental and physical health. Having understanding and helpful family and friends can be invaluable particularly as some carers may be reluctant to ask for support. Whilst there may not be any sign of appreciation of your efforts from the depressed person, support from family and friends can also suggest that the carer is a valued person. As one carer remarks:

'Compliments from friends and relatives - I never get any from the patient.'[5]

However, if family and friends are not aware of how severe depression can affect someone, they may say things which are likely to upset and annoy the depressed person such as 'you have a wonderful quality of life so how can you be feeling this way?' They may also suggest they should be putting more effort into getting themselves better. In addition, the depressed person may be concerned that some of the family and friends may gossip to others about their condition.

Trust and acceptance
Achieving a level of trust between you and the severely depressed person from the beginning of the illness may prove to be helpful.

Trust means that you and the depressed person have confidence in each other; that you will try and do your best for them and that they will be respected and listened to without being judged or criticized. Having trust in one another can be the fundamental basis needed for successful teamwork where you and the depressed person share common goals – the welfare and well-being of both. As one depressed person commented:

'If you trust someone ... you're half-way there.'[3]

Accepting that there is a limit to how much you can improve the person's condition for the better can also be helpful for the carer. In his book Speaking of Sadness, which details the effects of severe depression, David Karp tells of his appreciation for his wife's concern but also being upset at her incomprehension of his condition.

He describes his wife's eventual realization that:

'Nothing she could say or do would make much of a difference; even worse, that efforts to comfort me might only invite more negativity.'[6]

Carers find they have more peace of mind when they accept that:

'I did not cause it. I cannot control it. I cannot cure it. All I can do is cope with it.'[7]

PART 3 SEEKING HELP AND SUPPORT

There are things which you should now begin to do to gain help and support for yourself.

Early help and support is vital because the person's depression may last for some time and this could take a heavy toll on your own well-being. A useful first step is to talk to your GP to let them know that you are caring for someone with severe depression. This can be recorded on your medical records, and will help the GP to provide support to you when needed.

As there is little point stumbling along and learning on the job, it is the time when you need to talk to other people who are in similar circumstances.

In order to do this, you should consider contacting the local carers' advice centre as soon as possible in order to prepare and plan for the difficult times which may lie ahead. These centres are a good source for help, advice, understanding and support. Carers will appreciate that visiting these centres means they are able to speak to someone who listens.

Arrangements can also be made to meet and talk with other carers about how they are coping and which strategies they find works best. As some carers discovered:

'You need to be able to talk [about] what's going on with other people ... you need that respite in order to provide the right sort of support. Because I think every time you do that, you come back with a refreshed ... energy level and tolerance level.'[3]

'It's been so beneficial to me being involved in carers groups...just hearing everybody's story, and realising ...hang on – I'm not the only one going through this.'[3]

Quite often, the person experiencing the depression will be the one who generally deals with the bills and other financial matters. You might find yourself in the situation where the person with severe depression can no longer cope with this responsibility. Carer's centres can provide practical advice to help you before the situation begins to get out of hand.

Whilst learning from other carer's experiences and other sources can be helpful to some degree, the fact is that each severely depressed person experiences and reacts to the illness in their own individual way; a way which is unique to them. The same goes for the carer; the strategies employed and their reactions to situations can differ with each individual carer. Therefore, it is likely that what works best for one carer may not necessarily work for another, meaning that in certain cases, it may come down to you having to decide what works best by trial and error. As one carer discovered:

'it was a sort of trial and error, that's the way it felt to me ... So ... I don't know whether it's the right thing or not, well let's try it. Oh, it doesn't seem to work, well let's try something else.'[3]

There can even be cases where what is working best for you and the depressed person one day may not work the next day.

As one carer experienced:

'I could use the same techniques to try and deal with the situation that had ... worked perfectly the night before ... and get a completely different response.'[3]

Discovering new strategies which may work is one thing but seeking professional medical advice is another important step in getting the right treatment for the depressed person. However, there may be problems where for their own reasons, some people may be reluctant to seek treatment.

PART 4 STIGMA AND SEEKING TREATMENT

The stigma which surrounds severe depression is one of the main barriers that can make people reluctant to seek the treatment they need. It is likely that you will want them to seek professional help, and it can be difficult to encourage some people to do this because they fear being stigmatised.

They may feel embarrassed and ashamed and so wish to remain secretive about their illness. Some people may choose not to see their GP believing that it is an illness that they can handle themselves; think that it does not cause serious enough problems and not serious enough to seek treatment. There may also be worries that as their illness will go onto their medical record, it may prejudice their present or future employment. However, there are a number of organizations who are now very active in their anti-stigma campaigns for changing negative attitudes of the general public and employers. In recent times, a number of well known celebrities have been open about suffering from depression which has also gone a long way in de-stigmatizing the illness. Another issue can be their attitude to taking medication particularly antidepressants. Some people may have concerns about possible side effects associated with antidepressants and others believe that continued use will lead to addiction.

Persuading the person with severe depression to seek treatment

The importance of getting the earliest possible treatment is accurately summed up by the words of a depressed person who in hindsight admitted that:

'Everyone says 'but you look so well', you know, 'you look great', and 'there's nothing wrong, don't be silly', ... maybe if

I got help earlier, if someone had identified it and treated it more seriously, things would have been better.'[18]

The problem is now trying to persuade the person to agree that seeking treatment as soon as possible is a positive and necessary step towards recovery.

There can be ways in which you could gently persuade the reluctant person to seek treatment:

'If they don't seem to be bothering to get any kind of treatment, maybe a gentle reminder would do. They say that sometimes, people are more open to suggestions after they've thought about things for a while. And maybe if a bit more time goes by with nothing happening, another gentle reminder might work.'[19]

Perhaps making the point that if a severely depressed person is seriously interested in getting better, seeking medical advice and treatment can be an important step towards recovery.

When symptoms are less intensive, this could be one of the better opportunities to have a serious discussion about what you feel the person should do.

With symptoms of severe depression still persisting, the person has decided or been successfully persuaded by you that the time has come to visit the GP. If you can, it will always be helpful to accompany them.

On seeing the GP, the important thing is effective communication between the GP and the patient. There may be cases where severely depressed patients may have difficulty opening up to their GP to express their problems and emotions in a meaningful way. It may be difficult for the patient to explain what they are going through because severe depression is something of a mystery to them. They find it difficult to explain in words how they are feeling. However, you can have an important role to play in assisting the patient give the GP a full picture of what is happening especially as it is you who knows the patient best. In addition, severe depression can affect the patient's memory and you might find having to fill in the gaps in the story that the patient has forgotten to mention to the GP. In this way, you may improve the quality of care the patient receives from the GP. It is likely that when you are considered as a 'partner in care' by the GP, you may feel a greater source of purpose and importance which can help you feel more confident about your abilities and have more control of the situation.

Some patients frequently have concerns with taking up the GP's time. They may feel guilty that there are other patients waiting to see the GP and feel they have to rush their appointment. One patient sums this up well:
'It is as if you are making a fuss really ... and you don't have very long to actually speak to them, they have only got a certain time. So you haven't got enough time to actually,

you know, make them understand and for it to come across exactly how you feel.'[10]

But some GPs may recognize that the average consultation time is insufficient enough for a more detailed discussion with the patient and may offer another longer appointment. Being listened to by the GP is a major issue for patients. Patients place great value on a GP who is prepared to listen and show recognition and understanding of their condition. Patients believe that if listened to, they are being valued as a person and a sense that their problems are understood. Once the GP has diagnosed that the patient is suffering from severe depression, the next step is what form of treatment will be offered. In the majority of cases, GPs may decide on treatment with antidepressants as medical guidelines recommend this as first line treatment for severe depression. This is likely to send a message to the patient that they have no control over the illness which is something which has happened *to* them. The hope then is that the GP will prescribe a drug which will quickly cure the problem and that the drug will do all the work for them. However, some patients may have strong reservations about taking antidepressants and may prefer to try talking treatments first. If the GP decides that talking therapy is appropriate, they can refer the patient to a psychotherapist or counsellor. Cognitive behaviour therapy (CBT) is the common form of therapy. CBT sets out to help manage problems by changing the ways patients think and behave. Counselling is a type of psychological therapy and it involves the patient talking to a counsellor about their problems. Counsellors are trained to listen sympathetically and can help the patient deal with any negative thoughts and feelings.

However, there can sometimes be delays before the patient gets to see a therapist or counsellor but access to psychotherapy is slowly improving under the NHS programme: Improving Access to Psychological Therapies.

Confidentiality

Not all people want their carers to accompany them on their visit to the GP. One of the main barriers to a carer's knowledge of the patient's treatment by the GP can be the issue of confidentiality. The GP has a duty of confidentiality which means that what has been said and the treatments and advice given to the patient will not be revealed to the carer unless the patient agrees that the GP can share this information. There can be cases where the GP may be uneasy about sharing information with a carer and some may refuse to do so at all. But the GP should recognize that being excluded from the treatment process may make many carers feeling undervalued and irrelevant. However, carers who are sympathetic to the needs of the patient should be made to feel that they are part of the solution rather than the problem. Official guidelines for healthcare professionals state:

'Issues around confidentiality should not be used as a reason for not listening to carers, nor for not discussing fully with service users the need for carers to receive information so that they can continue to support them. Carers should be given sufficient information, in a way they can readily understand, to help them provide care efficiently.[11]

As a carer, you are entitled to see the GP on your own and raise any concerns you have about the patient and just as importantly, your own well-being.

'Carers indicate that ideally they and the person with the illness should be consulted independently as well as together. This is seen to greatly assist the carer with respect to management issues, yet allow the person with the illness to have privacy.'[12]

If the GP cannot inform the carer due to confidentiality, it may affect the quality of care the patient receives from the carer. If the GP believes the carer ought to be part of the treatment process, it is up to them to persuade the patient that it would be in their best interests to have the carer become more involved in the patient's welfare and treatment.

Medication and compliance

Because antidepressant treatment for severe depression is the rule rather than the exception, the issues surrounding whether the patient is taking medication as prescribed are important for both patient and carer. There are many brands of antidepressants available and individual GPs may have their own preferences and reasons for which drug they prescribe. It is also important to understand that all antidepressants are not the same; they work differently in the brain and so there may be cases where the first prescribed antidepressant may not be effective. If this is the case, the GP could switch to another brand. In any event, antidepressants can take up to 2 weeks to show any improvement but the full effect may take 4-6 weeks. It is important that the patient sticks to taking the antidepressant at the recommended dosage and at the recommended times. However, if the carer is not present at the consultation, not all patients may be willing to share details with the carer concerning the taking of their medication.

There is the danger that some patients may decide to stop taking them altogether because they feel better or take them when they feel the need to rather than sticking to the recommended daily dose. There have been cases where patients have taken more than the prescribed dosage wrongly believing it will have a quicker effect.

One of the main reasons for patients not continuing with medication is likely to be because of adverse side effects. Some patients may not be able to tolerate the side effects of the medication; feel worse and may decide to stop taking them. If this is the case, it is important that the patient should go back to their GP and tell them what has happened. Patient's attitudes towards taking antidepressant treatment may be influenced by what they have seen or read in the media and on websites regarding the possible adverse side effects of taking antidepressants. Much also rests on the information the GP has given to the patient; how long before the medication is likely to show any improvement in symptoms, explaining the benefits and possible adverse side effects and what might happen if the patient decides to discontinue the medication. As one patient experienced:

'I don't think there is enough explanation. I've seen three GPs and none of them actually explained what the tablets were that they were giving me. Just take them they'll make you feel better after a few weeks.'[13]

It has been noted that patients have more confidence in their treatment when the GP provided more detailed information about the nature and effects of antidepressants. This was more likely to lead to patients sticking to taking the medication as instructed by the GP.[13]

Not knowing how or if the patient is taking the medication may be a cause of concern for the carer. You may have reasons to suspect that the patient is not following the GP's instructions. But if there is an issue of confidentiality, how can the carer try to ensure that the patient is taking their medication in the right way?

The Royal College of Psychiatrists recognizes the role of the carer concerning medication by advising doctors that:

Very often the carer will have a role in assisting with medication compliancy and this role should be discussed and agreed with the carer. In such cases the carer needs full details of the medications, dosages and frequency of application. A copy of the care plan should be given to the carer wherever possible...

Despite this official advice, and due to the issue of confidentiality, the GP may still be prevented from involving the carer as part of the treatment team. In these circumstances, you could make an appointment with the GP to express your concerns that the patient is not following their advice.

PART 6 THE TREATMENT RESISTANT PATIENT

If the first prescribed antidepressant has no significant effect, the GP has the option of switching to a different brand but even this does not guarantee recovery. As the weeks pass and there are no signs of a reduction in symptoms, the patient may begin to lose faith in their GP's ability to cure them. With the medication not being effective, the loss of the patient's hope of a rapid recovery may deepen the depression to the point where the deteriorating patient may be considered as treatment resistant. This is likely to result in the patient being referred on to secondary care with a consultant psychiatrist. This would signal to the patient that they will be seeing an expert with the hope and expectation that they will be able to come up with a treatment that works. Psychiatrists through their specialized training have more detailed knowledge of severe depression and its treatments than GPs; they have the skills to prescribe new medication in addition to antidepressants that may be more successful. However, this means another wait to see if these new drugs will work. If you are able to accompany the patient, you can play an important role at this critical stage by reporting the behavioural patterns of the patient allowing the psychiatrist to have a more informed picture of the patient's condition and progress.

In cases where the medication is not working and there are signs that the patient may be seriously deteriorating further, the concerned psychiatrist may suggest to the patient that they should voluntarily go into hospital for a while so they are in constant observation and care. If the patient still shows no sign of improvement, as a last resort, the psychiatrist may suggest electroconvulsive therapy.

This is a treatment that can work for some and if it does, it can bring the patient out of the illness in a relatively short space of time. There are a number of issues regarding this particular treatment and the psychiatrist should fully inform the patient and just as importantly the carer of what to expect in terms of benefit and risk.

The effectiveness of the carer with the treatment resistant patient

Deep in to the illness and with no recovery in sight, the patient may begin to experience a deeper sense of hopelessness and become increasingly demoralized with their condition. They may become the least responsive to loving help and sympathy. It may be the case where your efforts to try and help the patient at this time is more likely to adversely affect you rather than improving the patient. It has been found that carers at this stage may become more stressed than at any time during the course of the patient's illness. Some carers may be at risk of becoming depressed themselves by this time. Although this may be difficult for you during this period, most carers decide that it is better to keep their feelings to themselves, especially anger thus avoiding worsening the patient's condition.[2] It is therefore important for you to have someone you can turn to for emotional support to help you through what is likely to be a challenging time.

Suicide

The longer time goes by without hope of recovery, there may be a risk that the patient may be seriously thinking about committing suicide. This is likely to become a major source of worry and concern for you.

Most people who suffer from severe depression will increasingly think about suicide at some point, and some may talk about their feelings but go no further than that. But if the patient and carer can talk openly about these suicidal thoughts and feelings, it can save a life. Begin by reassuring them that their life is very important to you, the family and close friends.

The Depression Alliance website offers the following advice:

Don't be afraid to ask them if they are suicidal, and try to reassure them that feeling or thinking the future is hopeless does not make it so in reality. If they have suicidal intentions, of have attempted suicide, call in other people (a GP, emergency services, social services) to help them and you with the situation. You can also contact The Samaritans.

However hard it may seem to look after a person who is suicidal, the fact that you are showing you care will have a positive impact.

Other than the carer, there may be cases where the psychiatrist may also detect that there is a serious risk of suicide and may decide to section the patient under the Mental Health Act meaning the patient is detained without their consent in a secure mental health hospital wing for observation.

PART 7 RECOVERY AND RELAPSE PREVENTION

Preventing a relapse back into severe depression after recovery is a very important issue. The last thing the patient and carer need after going through the first and difficult episode of severe depression is a return to another period of misery and stress.

Relapse prevention strategies can help patients avoid relapse altogether or have fewer and shorter episodes of the illness. Carers can be very important for assisting with many of the relapse prevention strategies and spotting early warning signs that the patient may be heading for a relapse.

Recovery is generally defined as the disappearance of the major symptoms for at least two consecutive months. The three items most frequently judged by patients to be very important in determining recovery were the presence of features of positive mental health such as optimism and self-confidence; a return to one's usual normal self and a return to usual level of functioning.[14] Other patients may still show an improvement but with signs of milder forms of symptoms still present. But in any event, the period of time after recovery and how it is managed is just as crucial for carer and patient as it was in the first episode of the illness.

There is a tendency for patients to believe that severe depression was an experience that had been overcome and will never be repeated. Some patients may be on a high and celebrating their recovery and may become over confident in their new found energy and start overdoing things which can result in them becoming stressed and fatigued. It is therefore important that carer and patient need to be aware that recovery is fragile and full recovery is an ongoing process. As many as 80% of recovered patients relapse between 6 to 9 months after recovery and remain vulnerable to further relapses for several years. With this high possibility of relapse, you need to be vigilant in recognizing when there are signs of symptoms returning.

One way of spotting early warning signs of possible relapse can be remembering the behaviour of the patient prior to the first episode of the illness and identifying any warning signs that were present at that time.

It may have needed a steady increase in levels of anxiety and an increase of negative thinking over a period of time to cause the slide into severe depression in the first place but after recovery, it can only take the faintest of triggers such as a person experiencing what would normally be considered as only a minor adverse event which could raise levels of anxiety and potentially lead in turn to another episode of severe depression. It is for this reason that once again, you can have a role to play in persuading the patient that it is important to receive effective ongoing treatment. Patients should continue on medication however, there is no guarantee that medication alone will prevent a relapse and other forms of treatment need to be in place. The patient may be still under the consultant psychiatrist at this stage. Because there is strong evidence suggesting that in addition to remaining on medication, psychotherapy is crucial in order to prevent a relapse, the psychiatrist should be referring and convincing the patient of the importance of receiving this form of treatment. CBT is the talking therapy that is the most often used but CBT may not suit everyone. There are a number of alternative talking therapies available. In any event, patients need good quality psychotherapy not only to get them better but also to teach them strategies how to stay that way.

However, some patients may initially have negative feelings towards psychotherapy; patients may feel it is too much of a struggle and lack the motivation to attend therapy sessions. Another issue is that the effectiveness of CBT or other talking therapies depends on the relationship which the patient and therapist are able to build with one another. Any therapy may not be effective if the therapist does not tailor the treatment to the needs of the individual patient and that patients may sense that they and the therapist are not on the same wavelength. Should this happen, it is likely to make the patient think, and with some justification, that attending further sessions would be pointless. However, it may be possible for the patient to switch therapists or type of therapy until the right one is found.

If affordable, another option could be to see a specialist therapist on a private basis. In any event, for any psychotherapy to be effective, the patient is likely to need a number of appointments. Psychotherapy will help the patient to make the necessary changes in their lifestyle and way of viewing what is important in their world in order to potentially reduce the risk and severity of relapse.

If a relapse does occur, perhaps the only source of comfort is that the duration of the relapse for some people can generally be much shorter than the first episode. It is also the time for you to remind the patient that they will recover as they did before.

The role of anxiety in relapse

It has been previously explained that anxiety and severe depression are strongly linked and that high levels of anxiety make severe depression a physically uncomfortable experience for many. After recovery from the first episode and for no apparent reason, symptoms of anxiety can strike without warning at any time even when things seem to be going well. Because some people associate the uncomfortable physical feelings of anxiety with severe depression, they may believe that they are heading for another episode of the illness. If this belief goes unchallenged, there is a serious risk of a slide back into severe depression.[15] Therefore, if you are aware that the person is experiencing this feeling, you could explain to them that it is more likely to be only a level of anxiety and once they realize this, it could help to change their attitude to the present situation and may help to prevent the slide into a full relapse.

PART 8 CARING FOR THE CARER

It is well recognized that carers need help and support to help them get through the almost relentless period of caring by maintaining their own health and well-being both mentally and physically. There are times where perhaps you should consider taking a step back from your situation and discover ways in which you could get back some of the enjoyment of living a happier life without totally abandoning the patient. As one carer began to realize:

'I have to take care of me. I'm important for myself and my family, too. I couldn't live my own life because I was too preoccupied with theirs. I told them, and I said, "I cried a tub full of tears and it never changed a thing." I still care. I care about them, but I cannot live like this, I mean live my life for them completely. That's too much you know.'[16]

You need to understand that you can only do so much and accept what can and can't be controlled. In order to avoid a physical and mental collapse, it is important to pace yourself by not trying to do too much because you may be caring for a lengthy period of time. Even if time is limited, doing something just for yourself will be helpful.

But if you are starting to experience problems with your own health due to high levels of stress, then this is the time for action. Visiting the GP is the first step. The GP may offer some form of treatment which can include referring you on to other healthcare professionals who offer talking therapies such as counsellors or psychotherapists. Carers may appreciate an opportunity to speak to a therapist who they can trust and where they can be more open about what they are going through. Other people that carers may find able to confide in and discuss their problems with would be sympathetic and understanding friends or relatives. Contacting the local carers' advice centre can also be helpful when things are becoming too much to handle. These centres provide helpful information on how carers can look after themselves: how the carer can attain a level of freedom, to have a life of their own and how to find time for themselves. Depending on circumstances, these advice centres can also organize ways for the carer to take a respite break away from their caring role.

There is growing recognition by the U.K. government of the contributions of carers. The *Department of Health Carers' Strategy 2008* includes a future commitment that: 'carers will be respected as expert carer partners and will have access to the integrated and personalised services they need to support them in their caring role', and that 'carers will be supported to stay mentally and physically well and treated with dignity'

PART 9 THE POSITIVES OF CARING

'I feel the capacity to care is the thing which gives life its deepest significance.'

Pablo Casals

The fact that you will be unable to completely lift the patient's depression may be the reality but that does not mean to say that you cannot make a positive difference that can benefit the patient. Good quality of care can help the recovery process; it can lead the patient to believe that they are cared for, loved and valued. It has also been found that in cases when carers are coping well in their role, the patient's depressive episode may last for a shorter period of time.[17]

Another important and positive example of the carer's value is that with the ever present risk of suicide in severe depression, carers can be life-savers. In comparison, patients who live alone have higher rates of attempted and completed suicide.

Research suggests carers who have a good sense of their own value and worth tend to interpret life events as positive challenges and these people also have the ability to find positive meaning to their role. Although there will always be some difficult times, carers can also learn from their experience by gaining an awareness of their inner strengths, becoming more self-confident, growing as a person, learning new things about themselves.[4]

Carers who can develop a positive appraisal and acceptance of the situation are more likely to suffer less stress and maintain a greater sense of competence, satisfaction and self-esteem.

It must also be remembered that severely depressed patients do eventually recover and this is another factor which can help keep you going through the really difficult times.

KEY POINTS TO REMEMBER

- Know the nature of severe depression and how it affects the patient

- Don't be alone – find all the help you can from understanding and sympathetic family and friends. Find advice and support from local carers organizations

- Encourage the patient to seek treatment

- Become involved as part of the treatment team with the help of the GP and other healthcare professionals

- Make time for yourself and look after your own health

- Accept that there is only so much you can do to help the patient to recovery

- Recovery is an ongoing process – be prepared for setbacks

- Try to encourage the patient to seek ongoing treatment after recovery